CODY SMITH

# One Exercise, 12 Weeks, Chiseled Abs

*Transform Your Core With This Sit-up Strength Training Workout Routine | at Home Workouts | No Gym Required |*

*First published by Nelaco Press 2021*

*Copyright © 2021 by Cody Smith*

*All rights reserved. No part of this publication may be reproduced, stored or transmitted in any form or by any means, electronic, mechanical, photocopying, recording, scanning, or otherwise without written permission from the publisher. It is illegal to copy this book, post it to a website, or distribute it by any other means without permission.*

*The exercises provided by the author (and the publisher) are for educational and entertainment purposes only, and are not to be interpreted as a recommendation for a specific course of action. Exercise is not without its risks, and this or any other exercise program may result in injury. They include but are not limited to: risk of injury, aggravation of a pre-existing condition, or adverse effect of over-exertion such as muscle strain, abnormal blood pressure, fainting, disorders of heartbeat, and very rare instances of heart attack. To reduce the risk of injury, before beginning this or any exercise program, please consult a healthcare provider for appropriate exercise prescription and safety precautions. The exercises instructions and advice presented are in no way intended as a substitute for medical consultation. The author (and the publisher) disclaims any liability from and in connection with this program. As with any exercise program, if at any point during your workout you begin to feel faint, dizzy, or have physical discomfort, you should stop immediately and consult a physician.*

*First edition*

*ISBN: 978-1-952381-21-8*

*This book was professionally typeset on Reedsy.
Find out more at reedsy.com*

# Contents

| | |
|---|---|
| *Preface* | viii |
| Before You Begin | 1 |
| Book 1 | 2 |
| Introduction: How to Use This Book | 3 |
| Initial Sit-up Assessment | 6 |
| Post-assessment Results | 8 |
| Completed Workouts Checklist | 10 |
| Completed Days Checklist | 11 |
| Pre and Post Challenge Measurements | 13 |
| Workout 1 | 14 |
| Workout 2 | 16 |
| Workout 3 | 18 |
| Workout 4 | 20 |
| Workout 5 | 22 |
| Workout 6 | 24 |
| Workout 7 | 26 |
| Workout 8 | 28 |
| Workout 9 | 30 |
| Workout 10 | 32 |
| Workout 11 | 34 |
| Workout 12 | 36 |
| Workout 13 | 38 |
| Workout 14 | 40 |
| Workout 15 | 42 |
| Workout 16 | 44 |
| Post 30 Day Assessment | 46 |

| | |
|---|---|
| Conclusion | 50 |
| Book 2 | 51 |
| Introduction - How to Use This Book | 52 |
| Initial Sit-up Assessment | 55 |
| Post-Assessment Results | 57 |
| Workout Completion Checklist | 60 |
| Pre & Post Program Measurements | 63 |
| Foundation Group Workouts | 64 |
| Foundation Group Workout 1 | 65 |
| Foundation Group Workout 2 | 66 |
| Foundation Group Workout 3 | 67 |
| Foundation Group Workout 4 | 68 |
| Foundation Group Workout 5 | 69 |
| Foundation Group Workout 6 | 70 |
| Novice Group Workouts | 71 |
| Novice Group Workout 1 | 72 |
| Novice Group Workout 2 | 73 |
| Novice Group Workout 3 | 74 |
| Novice Group Workout 4 | 76 |
| Novice Group Workout 5 | 77 |
| Novice Group Workout 6 | 78 |
| Newb Group Workouts | 80 |
| Newb Group Workout 1 | 81 |
| Newb Group Workout 2 | 82 |
| Newb Group Workout 3 | 83 |
| Newb Group Workout 4 | 85 |
| Newb Group Workout 5 | 86 |
| Newb Group Workout 6 | 87 |
| Greenhorn Group Workouts | 89 |
| Greenhorn Group Workout 1 | 90 |
| Greenhorn Group Workout 2 | 91 |
| Greenhorn Group Workout 3 | 92 |
| Greenhorn Group Workout 4 | 94 |

| | |
|---|---|
| Greenhorn Group Workout 5 | 95 |
| Greenhorn Group Workout 6 | 96 |
| Cub Group Workouts | 98 |
| Cub Group Workout 1 | 99 |
| Cub Group Workout 2 | 100 |
| Cub Group Workout 3 | 101 |
| Cub Group Workout 4 | 103 |
| Cub Group Workout 5 | 104 |
| Cub Group Workout 6 | 105 |
| Rookie Group Workouts | 107 |
| Rookie Group Workout 1 | 108 |
| Rookie Group Workout 2 | 109 |
| Rookie Group Workout 3 | 110 |
| Rookie Group Workout 4 | 112 |
| Rookie Group Workout 5 | 113 |
| Rookie Group Workout 6 | 114 |
| Pleb Group Workouts | 116 |
| Pleb Group Workout 1 | 117 |
| Pleb Group Workout 2 | 118 |
| Pleb Group Workout 3 | 119 |
| Pleb Group Workout 4 | 121 |
| Pleb Group Workout 5 | 122 |
| Pleb Group Workout 6 | 123 |
| Gorilla Group Workouts | 125 |
| Gorilla Group Workout 1 | 126 |
| Gorilla Group Workout 2 | 127 |
| Gorilla Group Workout 3 | 129 |
| Gorilla Group Workout 4 | 131 |
| Gorilla Group Workout 5 | 132 |
| Gorilla Group Workout 6 | 134 |
| Viking Group Workouts | 136 |
| Viking Group Workout 1 | 137 |
| Viking Group Workout 2 | 138 |

| | |
|---|---:|
| Viking Group Workout 3 | 140 |
| Viking Group Workout 4 | 142 |
| Viking Group Workout 5 | 143 |
| Viking Group Workout 6 | 145 |
| Elite Group Workouts | 147 |
| Elite Group Workout 1 | 148 |
| Elite Group Workout 2 | 149 |
| Elite Group Workout 3 | 151 |
| Elite Group Workout 4 | 153 |
| Elite Group Workout 5 | 154 |
| Elite Group Workout 6 | 156 |
| Commando Group Workouts | 158 |
| Commando Group Workout 1 | 159 |
| Commando Group Workout 2 | 160 |
| Commando Group Workout 3 | 162 |
| Commando Group Workout 4 | 164 |
| Commando Group Workout 5 | 165 |
| Commando Group Workout 6 | 167 |
| Veteran Group Workouts | 169 |
| Veteran Group Workout 1 | 170 |
| Veteran Group Workout 2 | 171 |
| Veteran Group Workout 3 | 173 |
| Veteran Group Workout 4 | 175 |
| Veteran Group Workout 5 | 176 |
| Veteran Group Workout 6 | 178 |
| Nuclear Group Workouts | 180 |
| Nuclear Group Workout 1 | 181 |
| Nuclear Group Workout 2 | 182 |
| Nuclear Group Workout 3 | 184 |
| Nuclear Group Workout 4 | 186 |
| Nuclear Group Workout 5 | 187 |
| Nuclear Group Workout 6 | 189 |
| Attempting 200 Consecutive Sit-ups | 191 |

Conclusion: 194

# Preface

Before you jump in and start knocking out more sit-ups than you have done in the past 3 years combined, I wanted to give a little guidance on how to use this book collection.

You are holding in your hands two books smashed into one to guide you for the next 12 weeks.

The first book is *300 Sit-ups a Day 30 Day Challenge*. The title says it all. These initial 30 days will give you a solid foundation to approach the second book, *8 Weeks to 200 Consecutive Sit-ups*.

I recommend going in order since the first book acts as a preparation phase to make sure you get the most out of the second book. At the end of the first book, you will complete a post 30-day assessment to see how many consecutive sit-ups you can put out. You can use the results from the first book as your initial sit-up assessment in the second book.

Having said that, you can absolutely skip the first book and head straight to the second if you want.

Your life. Your choice.

Also, do not forget to stretch out. Doing all these sit-ups can really do a number on your muscles and joints if you do not take time to properly recover.

Good luck.

**fist bump**

-Cody

# Before You Begin

Hey reader, thanks for grabbing a copy of the book.

If you are looking to pair this workout program with a complimentary guide to shed weight and boost your growth hormones to build more muscle faster, then I've got you covered.

Seems crazy to do both at the same time, but you can.

Better still, it is stupid easy.

Oh, and it is free. You can do this method anytime you want, anywhere for the rest of your life.

I usually sell this information, but I want you to have it.

You can get a copy from your cell phone from a simple text.

Seriously, get your phone out and text BOOST to (678) 506-7543.

Cheers!

# Book 1

300 Sit-ups a Day 30 Day Challenge

Workout Your Abs and Obliques While Developing a Better Posture and Stability With This Abdominal Exercise Program

By Cody Smith

# Introduction: How to Use This Book

Let me be the first to welcome you to the 300 sit-ups a day 30 day challenge program.

The next 30 days are going to be awesome as you work your way to completing literally 9000 sit-ups.

Sit-ups are a great, core engaging exercise that I truly believe is underrated.

Most people disregard sit-ups and dedicate time to countless ab crunches instead. Because sit-ups offer a wider range of motion, more muscles are targeted compared to a standard crunch.

Sit-ups help develop your core for higher levels of athletic performance, better balance, and stability.

Plus, they can be done practically anywhere you can anchor your feet.

Since this program is designed to be performed every single day, each workout is not focused on completely obliterating your abs to the point where you can't get out of bed the next morning.

Each workout is strategically designed to give you the optimum ratio of time your muscles are under tension and time your muscles are under rest so that you can perform it again the next day and not hate yourself.

The beginner workouts have less time under tension per set but take longer to complete the workout. The intermediate and advanced workouts have more time under tension making them significantly harder to perform but you are rewarded with a faster workout.

Before you wonder which workout to start with, I want you to know that there is zero guesswork required of where you need to start.

This program starts with an initial sit-up assessment to determine where you need to start in the program. Don't skip the assessment.

Once you complete the assessment, your 30 day challenge will start the very next day with whatever workout you're assigned from the post-assessment results.

While you're starting out in the program, you'll most likely be very sore early on in the program. Your body has not adapted to complete 300 sit-ups a day yet. That's okay, if the soreness is bearable, you can continue with the program.

If the soreness is unbearable, take a break for a few days until you recover and hop right back into the program where you left off.

If you can't complete your workout one day or have to skip a day here and there, don't fret. That's 300% okay and won't throw you way off. Quitting is the only failure.

Remember, this is a challenge. It's supposed to be challenging.

If it's too easy, the only thing you've gained is wasted time.

This brings me to the most important question:

## INTRODUCTION: HOW TO USE THIS BOOK

Are you ready to accept the challenge?

With that said, welcome to the 300 sit-ups a day challenge.

Head to the initial sit-up assessment and let the games begin.

# Initial Sit-up Assessment

Welcome to the initial sit-up assessment portion of this program. This is where we're going to check your current repetition count to see how many sit-ups you can actually perform without stopping.

This number will determine which workout you need to start with as you make your way through the 300 sit-up challenge program.

Make sure you are doing full sit-ups going all the way through the motion. Proper form is key to getting the most out of this exercise so I'll quickly go over how to properly perform a sit-up.

Lie on your back with knees bent at 90 degrees with your feet anchored. Tuck your chin into your neck or chest as you either interlace your fingers at the base of your skull or place both hands on the opposite upper chest/shoulder area. You will begin the exercise by lifting your upper body toward your thighs until your upper body is roughly perpendicular to the ground. Slowly lower your upper body back down to the floor to the point where your shoulder blades touch the ground before raising your upper body back up to complete the next rep.

It is important that you don't use your arms or heads to thrust your upper body toward your thighs. This is just cheating yourself out of doing a correct sit-up. All reps should be performed in a controlled manner.

## INITIAL SIT-UP ASSESSMENT

Go ahead complete as many sit-ups as you can without stopping using anything you want to anchor your feet.

When you're done, make note of how many you completed and head to the post-assessment results section.

# Post-assessment Results

Welcome to the post-assessment results section.

This is where you'll see what workout you'll start with based on the number of sit-ups you completed during the assessment.

Still got that number in your head?

Good.

- If you completed <18 sit-ups, your first workout starting tomorrow will be Workout 1.
- If you completed between 18 - 24 sit-ups, your first workout will be Workout 2.
- If you completed between 25 - 29 sit-ups, your first workout will be Workout 3.
- If you completed between 30 - 32 sit-ups, your first workout will be Workout 4.
- If you completed between 33 - 38 sit-ups, your first workout will be Workout 5.
- If you completed between 39 - 44 sit-ups, your first workout will be Workout 6.
- If you completed between 45 - 47sit-ups, your first workout will be

Workout 7.
- If you completed between 48 - 53 sit-ups, your first workout will be Workout 8.
- If you completed between 54 - 59 sit-ups, your first workout will be Workout 9.
- If you completed between 60 - 62 sit-ups, your first workout will be Workout 10.
- If you completed between 63 - 68 sit-ups, your first workout will be Workout 11.
- If you completed between 69 - 74 sit-ups, your first workout will be Workout 12.
- If you completed between 75 - 77 sit-ups, your first workout will be Workout 13.
- If you completed between 78 - 83 sit-ups, your first workout will be Workout 14.
- If you completed between 84 - 89 sit-ups, your first workout will be Workout 15.
- If you completed 90 or more sit-ups, your first workout will be Workout 16.

Don't fret if you didn't complete a lot of sit-ups. The point of the challenge is to start where you are and complete the full 30 days of 300 sit-ups a day. Not to be some amazing sit-up champion on day 1.

With that said, you know where you need to start starting tomorrow with your very first 300 sit-ups a day workout.

See you there.

# Completed Workouts Checklist

Check these off as you complete them:

_____Workout 1

_____Workout 2

_____Workout 3

_____Workout 4

_____Workout 5

_____Workout 6

_____Workout 7

_____Workout 8

_____Workout 9

_____Workout 10

_____Workout 11

_____Workout 12

_____Workout 13

_____Workout 14

_____Workout 15

_____Workout 16

# Completed Days Checklist

Date started: _____ (DD/MM/YYYY)

_____Day 1
_____Day 2
_____Day 3
_____Day 4
_____Day 5
_____Day 6
_____Day 7
_____Day 8
_____Day 9
_____Day 10
_____Day 11
_____Day 12
_____Day 13
_____Day 14
_____Day 15
_____Day 16
_____Day 17
_____Day 18
_____Day 19
_____Day 20
_____Day 21
_____Day 22
_____Day 23

_____Day 24
_____Day 25
_____Day 26
_____Day 27
_____Day 28
_____Day 29
_____Day 30

# Pre and Post Challenge Measurements

The following measurements are 100% optional and are not required to start or finish the program. I know some people will be curious to know other areas that are positively affected by completing the challenge.

Starting weight: _____

Starting sit-up rep max: _____

Starting timed plank hold max: _____

Ending weight: _____

Ending sit-up rep max: _____

Ending time plank hold max: _____

# Workout 1

Welcome to Workout 1 of the 300 sit-ups a day 30 day challenge.

For this workout, 3 sit-ups are performed every minute.

Because this is such a long workout, do your best to at least complete 50 sit-ups. Once you get stronger, re-do the initial assessment to work your way up the workout chain where the workouts are harder but take less time to complete.

This workout is way easier with an interval timer app. I suggest downloading one onto your phone with the following settings for this workout:

Intervals: 100

Time per interval: 1:06

That time will give you enough time to complete the number of correct sit-ups and enough time to rest between sets. The interval app also makes it easy to determine what set you're on.

With that said, go ahead and get started.

Come back in when you are done.

## WORKOUT 1

* * *

Way to go!

You completed 300 sit-ups today!

If that workout was too easy, consider moving up to the next workout.

If that workout was still fairly challenging, continue with this workout tomorrow.

That's all I've got for you today. See you tomorrow, champ!

# Workout 2

Welcome to Workout 2 of the 300 sit-ups a day 30 day challenge.

For this workout, 3 or 6 sit-ups are performed every minute.

The first 25 sets are 6 sit-ups each.

The last 50 sets are 3 sit-ups each.

Because this is such a long workout, do your best to at least complete 50 sit-ups. Once you get stronger, re-do the initial assessment to work your way up the workout chain where the workouts are harder but take less time to complete.

This workout is way easier with an interval timer app. I suggest downloading one onto your phone with the following settings for this workout:

Intervals: 75

Time per interval: 1:12

That time will give you enough time to complete the number of correct sit-ups and enough time to rest between sets. The interval app also makes it easy to determine what set you're on.

## WORKOUT 2

With that said, go ahead and get started.

Come back in when you are done.

* * *

Way to go!

You completed 300 sit-ups today!

If that workout was too easy, consider moving up to the next workout.

If that workout was still fairly challenging, continue with this workout tomorrow.

That's all I've got for you today. See you tomorrow, champ!

# Workout 3

Welcome to Workout 3 of the 300 sit-ups a day 30 day challenge.

For this workout, 3 or 6 sit-ups are performed every minute.

The first 40 sets are 6 sit-ups each.

The last 20 sets are 3 sit-ups each.

Because this is such a long workout, do your best to at least complete 50 sit-ups. Once you get stronger, re-do the initial assessment to work your way up the workout chain where the workouts are harder but take less time to complete.

This workout is way easier with an interval timer app. I suggest downloading one onto your phone with the following settings for this workout:

Intervals: 60

Time per interval: 1:12

That time will give you enough time to complete the number of correct sit-ups and enough time to rest between sets. The interval app also makes it easy to determine what set you're on.

WORKOUT 3

With that said, go ahead and get started.

Come back in when you are done.

*** 

Way to go!

You completed 300 sit-ups today!

If that workout was too easy, consider moving up to the next workout.

If that workout was still fairly challenging, continue with this workout tomorrow.

That's all I've got for you today. See you tomorrow, champ!

# Workout 4

Welcome to Workout 1 of the 300 sit-ups a day 30 day challenge.

For this workout, 6 sit-ups are performed every minute.

Because this is such a long workout, do your best to at least complete 50 sit-ups. Once you get stronger, re-do the initial assessment to work your way up the workout chain where the workouts are harder but take less time to complete.

This workout is way easier with an interval timer app. I suggest downloading one onto your phone with the following settings for this workout:

Intervals: 50

Time per interval: 1:12

That time will give you enough time to complete the number of correct sit-ups and enough time to rest between sets. The interval app also makes it easy to determine what set you're on.

With that said, go ahead and get started.

Come back in when you are done.

## WORKOUT 4

* * *

Way to go!

You completed 300 sit-ups today!

If that workout was too easy, consider moving up to the next workout.

If that workout was still fairly challenging, continue with this workout tomorrow.

That's all I've got for you today. See you tomorrow, champ!

# Workout 5

Welcome to Workout 5 of the 300 sit-ups a day 30 day challenge.

For this workout, 6 or 9 sit-ups are performed every minute.

The first 14 sets are 9 sit-ups each.

The last 29 sets are 6 sit-ups each.

This workout is way easier with an interval timer app. I suggest downloading one onto your phone with the following settings for this workout:

Intervals: 43

Time per interval: 1:18

That time will give you enough time to complete the number of correct sit-ups and enough time to rest between sets. The interval app also makes it easy to determine what set you're on.

With that said, go ahead and get started.

Come back in when you are done.

WORKOUT 5

*　*　*


Way to go!

You completed 300 sit-ups today!

If that workout was too easy, consider moving up to the next workout.

If that workout was still fairly challenging, continue with this workout tomorrow.

That's all I've got for you today. See you tomorrow, champ!

# Workout 6

Welcome to Workout 6 of the 300 sit-ups a day 30 day challenge.

For this workout, 6 or 9 sit-ups are performed every minute.

The first 24 sets are 9 sit-ups each.

The last 14 sets are 6 sit-ups each.

This workout is way easier with an interval timer app. I suggest downloading one onto your phone with the following settings for this workout:

Intervals: 38

Time per interval: 1:18

That time will give you enough time to complete the number of correct sit-ups and enough time to rest between sets. The interval app also makes it easy to determine what set you're on.

With that said, go ahead and get started.

Come back in when you are done.

## WORKOUT 6

\* \* \*

Way to go!

You completed 300 sit-ups today!

If that workout was too easy, consider moving up to the next workout.

If that workout was still fairly challenging, continue with this workout tomorrow.

That's all I've got for you today. See you tomorrow, champ!

# Workout 7

Welcome to Workout 7 of the 300 sit-ups a day 30 day challenge.

For this workout, 9 sit-ups are performed every minute.

The first 33 sets are 9 sit-ups each.

The last set is 3 sit-ups.

This workout is way easier with an interval timer app. I suggest downloading one onto your phone with the following settings for this workout:

Intervals: 34

Time per interval: 1:18

That time will give you enough time to complete the number of correct sit-ups and enough time to rest between sets. The interval app also makes it easy to determine what set you're on.

With that said, go ahead and get started.

Come back in when you are done.

## WORKOUT 7

* * *

Way to go!

You completed 300 sit-ups today!

If that workout was too easy, consider moving up to the next workout.

If that workout was still fairly challenging, continue with this workout tomorrow.

That's all I've got for you today. See you tomorrow, champ!

# Workout 8

Welcome to Workout 8 of the 300 sit-ups a day 30 day challenge.

For this workout, 9 or 12 sit-ups are performed every minute.

The first 10 sets are 12 sit-ups each.

The last 20 sets are 9 sit-ups each.

This workout is way easier with an interval timer app. I suggest downloading one onto your phone with the following settings for this workout:

Intervals: 30

Time per interval: 1:24

That time will give you enough time to complete the number of correct sit-ups and enough time to rest between sets. The interval app also makes it easy to determine what set you're on.

With that said, go ahead and get started.

Come back in when you are done.

# WORKOUT 8

\* \* \*

Way to go!

You completed 300 sit-ups today!

If that workout was too easy, consider moving up to the next workout.

If that workout was still fairly challenging, continue with this workout tomorrow.

That's all I've got for you today. See you tomorrow, champ!

# Workout 9

Welcome to Workout 9 of the 300 sit-ups a day 30 day challenge.

For this workout, 9 or 12 sit-ups are performed every minute.

The first 18 sets are 12 sit-ups each.

The next 9 sets are 9 sit-ups each.

The last set is 3 sit-ups.

This workout is way easier with an interval timer app. I suggest downloading one onto your phone with the following settings for this workout:

Intervals: 28

Time per interval: 1:24

That time will give you enough time to complete the number of correct sit-ups and enough time to rest between sets. The interval app also makes it easy to determine what set you're on.

With that said, go ahead and get started.

## WORKOUT 9

Come back in when you are done.

* * *

Way to go!

You completed 300 sit-ups today!

If that workout was too easy, consider moving up to the next workout.

If that workout was still fairly challenging, continue with this workout tomorrow.

That's all I've got for you today. See you tomorrow, champ!

# Workout 10

Welcome to Workout 10 of the 300 sit-ups a day 30 day challenge.

For this workout, 12 sit-ups are performed every minute.

This workout is way easier with an interval timer app. I suggest downloading one onto your phone with the following settings for this workout:

Intervals: 25

Time per interval: 1:24

That time will give you enough time to complete the number of correct sit-ups and enough time to rest between sets. The interval app also makes it easy to determine what set you're on.

With that said, go ahead and get started.

Come back in when you are done.

* * *

## WORKOUT 10

Way to go!

You completed 300 sit-ups today!

If that workout was too easy, consider moving up to the next workout.

If that workout was still fairly challenging, continue with this workout tomorrow.

That's all I've got for you today. See you tomorrow, champ!

# Workout 11

Welcome to Workout 11 of the 300 sit-ups a day 30 day challenge.

For this workout, 12 or 15 sit-ups are performed every minute.

The first 8 sets are 15 sit-ups each.

The last 15 sets are 12 sit-ups each.

This workout is way easier with an interval timer app. I suggest downloading one onto your phone with the following settings for this workout:

Intervals: 23

Time per interval: 1:30

That time will give you enough time to complete the number of correct sit-ups and enough time to rest between sets. The interval app also makes it easy to determine what set you're on.

With that said, go ahead and get started.

Come back in when you are done.

## WORKOUT 11

* * *

Way to go!

You completed 300 sit-ups today!

If that workout was too easy, consider moving up to the next workout.

If that workout was still fairly challenging, continue with this workout tomorrow.

That's all I've got for you today. See you tomorrow, champ!

# Workout 12

Welcome to Workout 12 of the 300 sit-ups a day 30 day challenge.

For this workout, 12 or 15 sit-ups are performed every minute.

The first 14 sets are 15 sit-ups each.

The next 7 sets are 12 sit-ups each.

The last set is 6 sit-ups.

This workout is way easier with an interval timer app. I suggest downloading one onto your phone with the following settings for this workout:

Intervals: 22

Time per interval: 1:30

That time will give you enough time to complete the number of correct sit-ups and enough time to rest between sets. The interval app also makes it easy to determine what set you're on.

With that said, go ahead and get started.

# WORKOUT 12

Come back in when you are done.

*** 

Way to go!

You completed 300 sit-ups today!

If that workout was too easy, consider moving up to the next workout.

If that workout was still fairly challenging, continue with this workout tomorrow.

That's all I've got for you today. See you tomorrow, champ!

# Workout 13

Welcome to Workout 13 of the 300 sit-ups a day 30 day challenge.

For this workout, 15 sit-ups are performed every minute.

This workout is way easier with an interval timer app. I suggest downloading one onto your phone with the following settings for this workout:

Intervals: 20

Time per interval: 1:30

That time will give you enough time to complete the number of correct sit-ups and enough time to rest between sets. The interval app also makes it easy to determine what set you're on.

With that said, go ahead and get started.

Come back in when you are done.

\* \* \*

Way to go!

You completed 300 sit-ups today!

If that workout was too easy, consider moving up to the next workout.

If that workout was still fairly challenging, continue with this workout tomorrow.

That's all I've got for you today. See you tomorrow, champ!

# Workout 14

Welcome to Workout 14 of the 300 sit-ups a day 30 day challenge.

For this workout, 15 or 18 sit-ups are performed every minute.

The first 6 sets are 18 sit-ups each.

The next 12 sets are 15 sit-ups each.

The last set is 12 sit-ups.

This workout is way easier with an interval timer app. I suggest downloading one onto your phone with the following settings for this workout:

Intervals: 19

Time per interval: 1:36

That time will give you enough time to complete the number of correct sit-ups and enough time to rest between sets. The interval app also makes it easy to determine what set you're on.

With that said, go ahead and get started.

## WORKOUT 14

Come back in when you are done.

$$* * *$$

Way to go!

You completed 300 sit-ups today!

If that workout was too easy, consider moving up to the next workout.

If that workout was still fairly challenging, continue with this workout tomorrow.

That's all I've got for you today. See you tomorrow, champ!

# Workout 15

Welcome to Workout 15 of the 300 sit-ups a day 30 day challenge.

For this workout, 15 or 18 sit-ups are performed every minute.

The first 11 sets are 18 sit-ups each.

The next 6 sets are 15 sit-ups each.

The last set is 12 sit-ups.

This workout is way easier with an interval timer app. I suggest downloading one onto your phone with the following settings for this workout:

Intervals: 18

Time per interval: 1:36

That time will give you enough time to complete the number of correct sit-ups and enough time to rest between sets. The interval app also makes it easy to determine what set you're on.

With that said, go ahead and get started.

## WORKOUT 15

Come back in when you are done.

* * *

Way to go!

You completed 300 sit-ups today!

If that workout was too easy, consider moving up to the next workout.

If that workout was still fairly challenging, continue with this workout tomorrow.

That's all I've got for you today. See you tomorrow, champ!

# Workout 16

Welcome to Workout 16 of the 300 sit-ups a day 30 day challenge.

For this workout, 18 sit-ups are performed every minute.

The first 16 sets are 18 sit-ups each.

The last set is 12 sit-ups.

This workout is way easier with an interval timer app. I suggest downloading one onto your phone with the following settings for this workout:

Intervals: 17

Time per interval: 1:36

That time will give you enough time to complete the number of correct sit-ups and enough time to rest between sets. The interval app also makes it easy to determine what set you're on.

With that said, go ahead and get started.

Come back in when you are done.

## WORKOUT 16

* * *

Way to go!

You completed 300 sit-ups today!

That's more than most people do in a year.

That's all I've got for you today. See you tomorrow, champ!

# Post 30 Day Assessment

Hey champ, before we get into the post-assessment, I'd like to ask you for a quick favor.

I'm going to be greedy for a minute here and ask you to leave a review for the book.

Maybe give a star for every time your entire body shook from trying to complete a sit-up.

Reviews are a pain to get but it'll only take a minute or two to leave one.

So while you're warming up to destroy this assessment, pull your phone out and scan this QR code.

## POST 30 DAY ASSESSMENT

It'll take you straight to the book's page on Amazon.

Scroll to the bottom and click 'Leave a Customer Review.' Leave a star rating, say a few words, and click submit.

It's that simple!

Once you're done, come back to crush your assessment.

You accepted the 30 day challenge, you completed the 30 day challenge, and now it's time to see where you are now after nailing down 9000 sit-ups.

This is pretty exciting.

All that hard work, dedication, and blisters to get to this point.

I hope to goodness sake you've allowed a couple of days to recover between the 30th day of your challenge and now.

You'll see much better results that way.

With that said, get ready to crush this assessment.

Remember that number you started out with during the first assessment?

Go ahead and say that number out loud.

You're about to blow past that number.

Go ahead complete as many sit-ups as you can without stopping.

\* \* \*

How'd you do?

Satisfied with your new number?

## POST 30 DAY ASSESSMENT

Yes and no right?

Yes because you knocked out way more reps and no because you're hungry for more!

Don't be afraid to take a week off and start the challenge again with your new assessment number.

# Conclusion

Hey champ, I really hope you enjoyed the 300 sit-ups a day 30 day program.

I hope it was challenging, I hope you pushed yourself, and I hope your post-assessment was worthy of a killer high five.

If you're thirsty for more challenges, we've got more where this came from.

And if you've enjoyed this book, do take a second to leave a review.

Those jokers are hard to get but will only take a minute or two for you to leave one.

Until next time, champ.

# Book 2

8 Weeks to 200 Consecutive Sit-ups

Build a Strong Core by Working Your Abs, Obliques, and Lower Back
| at Home Workouts | No Gym Required |

By Cody Smith

# Introduction - How to Use This Book

If you asked random people on the street how to get six-pack abs, they would probably tell you to do crunches.

Sure, they work your abs but not like sit-ups.

Sit-ups work your entire core when done correctly, but you would see a whole lot of people doing them in the gym.

You will find people working on workout equipment for hours when all they need is their body to get the job done.

And you would be hard-pressed to find a lot of people even in a gym who can do even 50 consecutive sit-ups.

But we are not here to shoot for a mere 50. We are going straight for 200 consecutive smackeroos.

We are hitting 3 digits here or we are going home. All or nothing baby.

And that's exactly what you're going to find here in this 8-week program.

Sure, you could do sit-ups on your own, try and knock out as many as possible every day and work your way to 200 but you are either going to fall short or give up before you even get there.

## INTRODUCTION - HOW TO USE THIS BOOK

What you need is strategically designed workouts for your current fitness level that challenge you just enough without killing you. Each workout will push you for the proper progression to make steady gains along the way. This program is structured to take all the guesswork out of your journey to 200 consecutive sit-ups.

And these workouts can literally be completed anywhere as long as you have somewhere, something, or someone to anchor your feet.

Your journey begins with an initial sit-up assessment to find out where your current max is. Afterward, you will know exactly where to start in the program.

Once you complete the entire program, you will have earned the right to attempt nailing 200 consecutive sit-ups.

Some people knock it out on their first try. Others will not and will need to hack it a few more weeks before trying again.

Now, I will warn you, these workouts can feel very repetitive at times. Far too often people look for variety and complexity to see results when really the simplest of approaches is best.

100 sit-ups variations and off-the-wall workout routines are not what is going to get you to the results you want. Showing up and putting in the work; that is where the real bacon is.

Some of you will not need the entire 8 weeks. Others will need more than 8 weeks. Either way is perfectly fine and doesn't mean the program doesn't work, it just means everyone comes from a different level of fitness.

8 weeks is not some magical number that will work for every single person. 8 weeks is the average amount of time it will take the average person to reach

200 consecutive sit-ups so do not get too caught up in the timeline. It will take you however long that it takes you.

What I can promise you is if you put in the work, you will see the results.

Up next is the initial assessment. Get after it, champ.

# Initial Sit-up Assessment

This is the first step into your incredible journey to doing 200 consecutive sit-ups. It will be hard but manageable as you embark on something that very few people on the face of the earth have ever accomplished.

We are going to start out with a sit-up assessment to determine where you should start in the program.

Make sure you are doing full sit-ups going all the way through the motion. Proper form is key to getting the most out of this exercise, so I'll quickly go over how to properly perform a sit-up.

Lie on your back with knees bent at 90 degrees with your feet anchored. Tuck your chin into your neck or chest as you either interlace your fingers at the base of your skull or place both hands on the opposite upper chest/shoulder area. You will begin the exercise by lifting your upper body toward your thighs until your upper body is roughly perpendicular to the ground. Slowly lower your upper body back down to the floor to the point where your shoulder blades touch the ground before raising your upper body back up to complete the next rep.

It is important that you do not use your arms or heads to thrust your upper body toward your thighs. This is just cheating yourself out of doing a correct sit-up. All reps should be performed in a controlled manner.

Go ahead and complete as many correct sit-ups as you can without stopping using something sturdy to anchor your feet like a toe bar, couch, or dresser.

Once you are done, remember the number of fully-completed sit-ups and head to the post-assessment results section.

Note: If this is the first assessment, you will write your assessment number in the '1st assessment' row. When you come back to do another assessment, you write in your completed number of reps in the respective row depending on how many assessments you have completed.

_____ reps: 1st assessment
_____ reps: 2nd assessment
_____ reps: 3rd assessment
_____ reps: 4th assessment
_____ reps: 5th assessment
_____ reps: 6th assessment
_____ reps: 7th assessment
_____ reps: 8th assessment
_____ reps: 9th assessment
_____ reps: 10th assessment
_____ reps: 11th assessment
_____ reps: 12th assessment
_____ reps: 13th assessment
_____ reps: 14th assessment
_____ reps: 15th assessment
_____ reps: 16th assessment
_____ reps: 17th assessment
_____ reps: 18th assessment
_____ reps: 19th assessment
_____ reps: 20th assessment

# Post-Assessment Results

So... how did you do?

Were you surprised with how many you did or were you underwhelmed and disappointed that you did not do so hot?

Do not beat yourself up. This is simply a baseline for you to start from.

Go ahead and jog your memory of your assessment score.

With that score in mind, you are now going to be directed to your workout grouping based on your score.

Do not get too caught up in the name of each group of workouts, these are just fun names to identify which group you are currently in. If you do not like your current group name, do not worry, stick with the program long enough and you will be out of that group in no time and into another group whose name you probably will not like either.

Before I go into informing you of your baseline workout, I recommend leaving a day between now and hitting your first workout to recover from your assessment. However, you do not have to if you are feeling gung-ho and want to go ahead and knock out your first workout.

- If you did less than 10, you will start in the Foundation Group to build up your strength.
- If you did 10, you will start in the Novice Group.
- If you did between 11 and 20, you will start in the Newb Group.
- If you did between 21 and 30, you will start in the Greenhorn Group.
- If you did between 31 and 40, you will start in the Cub Group.
- If you did between 41 and 50, you will start in the Rookie Group.
- If you did between 51 and 60, you will start in the Pleb Group.
- If you did between 61 and 70, you will start in the Gorilla Group.
- If you did between 71 and 80, you will start in the Viking Group.
- If you did between 81 and 90, you will start in the Elite Group.
- If you did between 91 and 100, you will start in the Commando Group.
- If you did between 101 and 110, you will start in the Veteran Group.
- If you did greater than 110, you will start in the Nuclear Group.

Now that you know your group, you know where you will begin for your next workout.

In your group, you will start with workout 1 followed by workout 2 and 3.

For example, let's say you completed 23 reps, and you were going to workout Monday, Wednesday, and Friday. That would put you in the Greenhorn Group with workout 1 on Monday, Workout 2 on Wednesday, and workout 3 on Friday.

The following week, you would start with greenhorn Group Workout 4 followed by 5 and 6.

Simple enough.

Also, some of your workouts will involve what I call fundamental sit-ups.

Fundamental sit-ups involve a very slow descend and a normal ascend during the sit-up exercise. These work the full range of muscles throughout the entire sit-ups. Typical sit-ups only provide significant tensions when you raise your body from the floor. These sit-ups make you work during the descent and the rise. You will have either 5 or 10 second descends during your workouts.

For example, if you have a set of 3 fundamental sit-ups with 5 seconds descends, you will start in the up, ready position and lower yourself slowly over a 5 second period to the bottom of the exercise when your shoulder blades touch the floor. You will then pull back up to the starting position like a normal sit-up. As soon as you get to the top of the exercise, you will begin gradually lowering yourself back down over another 5 second period for the second rep followed by the third.

They do not sound bad, but boy do they start to burn quick.

Great job on your assessment and get ready for your first workout.

# Workout Completion Checklist

Check off your workouts as you complete them:
- _____Foundation Group Workout 1
- _____Foundation Group Workout 2
- _____Foundation Group Workout 3
- _____Foundation Group Workout 4
- _____Foundation Group Workout 5
- _____Foundation Group Workout 6
- _____Novice Group Workout 1
- _____Novice Group Workout 2
- _____Novice Group Workout 3
- _____Novice Group Workout 4
- _____Novice Group Workout 5
- _____Novice Group Workout 6
- _____Newb Group Workout 1
- _____Newb Group Workout 2
- _____Newb Group Workout 3
- _____Newb Group Workout 4
- _____Newb Group Workout 5
- _____Newb Group Workout 6
- _____Greenhorn Group Workout 1
- _____Greenhorn Group Workout 2
- _____Greenhorn Group Workout 3
- _____Greenhorn Group Workout 4
- _____Greenhorn Group Workout 5

## WORKOUT COMPLETION CHECKLIST

_____Greenhorn Group Workout 6
_____Cub Group Workout 1
_____Cub Group Workout 2
_____Cub Group Workout 3
_____Cub Group Workout 4
_____Cub Group Workout 5
_____Cub Group Workout 6
_____Rookie Group Workout 1
_____Rookie Group Workout 2
_____Rookie Group Workout 3
_____Rookie Group Workout 4
_____Rookie Group Workout 5
_____Rookie Group Workout 6
_____Pleb Group Workout 1
_____Pleb Group Workout 2
_____Pleb Group Workout 3
_____Pleb Group Workout 4
_____Pleb Group Workout 5
_____Pleb Group Workout 6
_____Gorilla Group Workout 1
_____Gorilla Group Workout 2
_____Gorilla Group Workout 3
_____Gorilla Group Workout 4
_____Gorilla Group Workout 5
_____Gorilla Group Workout 6
_____Viking Group Workout 1
_____Viking Group Workout 2
_____Viking Group Workout 3
_____Viking Group Workout 4
_____Viking Group Workout 5
_____Viking Group Workout 6
_____Elite Group Workout 1
_____Elite Group Workout 2

_____Elite Group Workout 3
_____Elite Group Workout 4
_____Elite Group Workout 5
_____Elite Group Workout 6
_____Commando Group Workout 1
_____Commando Group Workout 2
_____Commando Group Workout 3
_____Commando Group Workout 4
_____Commando Group Workout 5
_____Commando Group Workout 6
_____Veteran Group Workout 1
_____Veteran Group Workout 2
_____Veteran Group Workout 3
_____Veteran Group Workout 4
_____Veteran Group Workout 5
_____Veteran Group Workout 6
_____Nuclear Group Workout 1
_____Nuclear Group Workout 2
_____Nuclear Group Workout 3
_____Nuclear Group Workout 4
_____Nuclear Group Workout 5
_____Nuclear Group Workout 6
_____Attempting 200 Consecutive Sit-ups
_____Completed 200 Consecutive Sit-ups: _____ reps.

# Pre & Post Program Measurements

The following measurements are 100% optional and are not required to start or finish the program. I know some people will be curious to know other areas that are positively affected by achieving 200 consecutive sit-ups.

Starting weight: _____

Starting sit-up rep max: _____

Starting timed plank hold max: _____

Ending weight: _____

Ending sit-up rep max: _____

Ending time plank hold max: _____

# Foundation Group Workouts

# Foundation Group Workout 1

Welcome to the Foundation Group Workout 1.

For this workout, you have 5 sets with 60 seconds of rest between each set consisting of negative sit-ups.

Negative sit-ups simply focus on a slow descent without ascending to the up position. This means as soon as you complete your descent, you can stop and rest.

Go ahead and get into the starting position with your feet anchored in the up, ready position, upper body perpendicular to the floor.

Sets:

1. 1 negative sit-up with a 3 second descend.
2. 1 negative sit-up with a 3 second descend.
3. 1 negative sit-up with a 3 second descend.
4. 1 negative sit-up with a 3 second descend.
5. 1 negative sit-up with a 3 second descend.

If you completed this workout, head to Foundation Group Workout 2 for your next session. If not, stick with this one until you complete it.

# Foundation Group Workout 2

Welcome to the Foundation Group Workout 2.

For this workout, you have 5 sets with 60 seconds of rest between each set consisting of negative sit-ups.

Remember to focus on proper form throughout your sets and always start in the up, ready position.

Sets:

1. 1 negative sit-up with a 3 second descend.
2. 1 negative sit-up with a 5 second descend.
3. 1 negative sit-up with a 5 second descend.
4. 1 negative sit-up with a 3 second descend.
5. 1 negative sit-up with a 3 second descend.

If you completed this workout, head to Foundation Group Workout 3 for your next session. If not, stick with this one until you complete it.

# Foundation Group Workout 3

Welcome to the Foundation Group Workout 3.

For this workout, you have 5 sets with 60 seconds of rest between each set consisting of negative sit-ups.

Remember to focus on proper form throughout your sets and always start in the up, ready position.

Sets:

1. 1 negative sit-up with a 5 second descend.
2. 1 negative sit-up with a 5 second descend.
3. 1 negative sit-up with a 5 second descend.
4. 1 negative sit-up with a 5 second descend.
5. 1 negative sit-up with a 5 second descend.

If you completed this workout, head to Foundation Group Workout 4 for your next session. If not, stick with this one until you complete it.

# Foundation Group Workout 4

Welcome to the Foundation Group Workout 4.

For this workout, you have 5 sets with 60 seconds of rest between each set consisting of negative sit-ups.

Remember to focus on proper form throughout your sets and always start in the up, ready position.

Sets:

1. 1 negative sit-up with a 5 second descend.
2. 1 negative sit-up with a 5 second descend.
3. 1 negative sit-up with a 7 second descend.
4. 1 negative sit-up with a 7 second descend.
5. 1 negative sit-up with a 7 second descend.

If you completed this workout, head to Foundation Group Workout 5 for your next session. If not, stick with this one until you complete it.

# Foundation Group Workout 5

Welcome to the Foundation Group Workout 5.

For this workout, you have 5 sets with 60 seconds of rest between each set consisting of negative sit-ups.

Remember to focus on proper form throughout your sets and always start in the up, ready position.

Sets:

1. 1 negative sit-up with a 7 second descend.
2. 1 negative sit-up with a 7 second descend.
3. 1 negative sit-up with a 7 second descend.
4. 1 negative sit-up with a 7 second descend.
5. 1 negative sit-up with a 7 second descend.

If you completed this workout, head to Foundation Group Workout 6 for your next session. If not, stick with this one until you complete it.

# Foundation Group Workout 6

Welcome to the Foundation Group Workout 6.

For this workout, you have 5 sets with 60 seconds of rest between each set consisting of negative sit-ups.

Remember to focus on proper form throughout your sets and always start in the up, ready position.

Sets:

1. 1 negative sit-up with a 10 second descend.
2. 1 negative sit-up with a 10 second descend.
3. 1 negative sit-up with a 10 second descend.
4. 1 negative sit-up with a 10 second descend.
5. 1 negative sit-up with a 10 second descend.

Since this is the end of a two-week period, it is time to redo your sit-up assessment to check your progress. Rest a day and give the assessment a go to see which Group you will be in next.

# Novice Group Workouts

# Novice Group Workout 1

Welcome to the Novice Group Workout 1.

For this workout, you have 6 sets with 60 seconds of rest between each set.

Remember to focus on proper form throughout your sets.

Sets:

1. 5 sit-ups
2. 5 sit-ups
3. 5 sit-ups
4. 5 sit-ups
5. 5 sit-ups
6. 1 fundamental sit-up with a 5 second descend.

If you completed this workout, head to Novice Group Workout 2 for your next session. If not, stick with this one until you complete it.

Glasses of water drank today: 1-2-3-4-5-6-7-8-9-10

Hours of sleep last night: 1-2-3-4-5-6-7-8-9-10

Diet: junk: junk food —————semi-healthy—————healthy

# Novice Group Workout 2

Welcome to the Novice Group Workout 2.

For this workout, you have 6 sets with 60 seconds of rest between each set.

Remember to focus on proper form throughout your sets.

Sets:

1. 7 sit-ups
2. 7 sit-ups
3. 7 sit-ups
4. 7 sit-ups
5. 7 sit-ups
6. 2 fundamental sit-ups with a 5 second descend.

If you completed this workout, head to Novice Group Workout 3 for your next session. If not, stick with this one until you complete it.

Glasses of water drank today: 1-2-3-4-5-6-7-8-9-10

Hours of sleep last night: 1-2-3-4-5-6-7-8-9-10

Diet: junk: junk food—————semi-healthy—————healthy

# Novice Group Workout 3

Welcome to the Novice Group Workout 3.

For this workout, you have 6 sets with 90 seconds of rest between each set.

Remember to focus on proper form throughout your sets.

Sets:

1. 8 sit-ups
2. 8 sit-ups
3. 8 sit-ups
4. 8 sit-ups
5. 8 sit-ups
6. Max out: perform as many sit-ups as you can.

Max reps: _____

If you completed this workout, head to Novice Group Workout 4 for your next session. If not, stick with this one until you complete it.

Glasses of water drank today: 1-2-3-4-5-6-7-8-9-10

Hours of sleep last night: 1-2-3-4-5-6-7-8-9-10

Diet: junk: junk food—————semi-healthy—————healthy

# Novice Group Workout 4

Welcome to the Novice Group Workout 4.

For this workout, you have 6 sets with 60 seconds of rest between each set.

Remember to focus on proper form throughout your sets.

Sets:

1. 10 sit-ups
2. 10 sit-ups
3. 10 sit-ups
4. 10 sit-ups
5. 10 sit-ups
6. 3 fundamental sit-ups with a 5 second descend.

If you completed this workout, head to Novice Group Workout 5 for your next session. If not, stick with this one until you complete it.

Glasses of water drank today: 1-2-3-4-5-6-7-8-9-10

Hours of sleep last night: 1-2-3-4-5-6-7-8-9-10

Diet: junk: junk food—————semi-healthy—————healthy

# Novice Group Workout 5

Welcome to the Novice Group Workout 5.

For this workout, you have 6 sets with 60 seconds of rest between each set.

Remember to focus on proper form throughout your sets.

Sets:

1. 11 sit-ups
2. 11 sit-ups
3. 11 sit-ups
4. 11 sit-ups
5. 11 sit-ups
6. 3 fundamental sit-ups with a 5 second descend.

If you completed this workout, head to Novice Group Workout 6 for your next session. If not, stick with this one until you complete it.

Glasses of water drank today: 1-2-3-4-5-6-7-8-9-10

Hours of sleep last night: 1-2-3-4-5-6-7-8-9-10

Diet: junk: junk food—————semi-healthy—————healthy

# Novice Group Workout 6

Welcome to the Novice Group Workout 6.

For this workout, you have 6 sets with 90 seconds of rest between each set.

Remember to focus on proper form throughout your sets.

Sets:

1. 14 sit-ups
2. 14 sit-ups
3. 14 sit-ups
4. 14 sit-ups
5. 14 sit-ups
6. Max out: perform as many sit-ups as you can.

Max reps: _____

Since this is the end of a two-week period, it is time to redo your sit-up assessment to check your progress if you fully completed this workout.

Rest a day and give the assessment a go to see which Group you will be in next.

## NOVICE GROUP WORKOUT 6

Glasses of water drank today: 1-2-3-4-5-6-7-8-9-10

Hours of sleep last night: 1-2-3-4-5-6-7-8-9-10

Diet: junk: junk food—————semi-healthy—————healthy

# Newb Group Workouts

# Newb Group Workout 1

Welcome to the Newb Group Workout 1.

For this workout, you have 6 sets with 60 seconds of rest between each set.

Remember to focus on proper form throughout your sets.

Sets:

1. 11 sit-ups
2. 11 sit-ups
3. 11 sit-ups
4. 11 sit-ups
5. 11 sit-ups
6. 2 fundamental sit-ups with a 5 second descend.

If you completed this workout, head to Newb Group Workout 2 for your next session. If not, stick with this one until you complete it.

Glasses of water drank today: 1-2-3-4-5-6-7-8-9-10

Hours of sleep last night: 1-2-3-4-5-6-7-8-9-10

Diet: junk: junk food—————semi-healthy—————healthy

# Newb Group Workout 2

Welcome to the Newb Group Workout 2.

For this workout, you have 6 sets with 60 seconds of rest between each set.

Remember to focus on proper form throughout your sets.

Sets:

1. 14 sit-ups
2. 14 sit-ups
3. 14 sit-ups
4. 14 sit-ups
5. 14 sit-ups
6. 3 fundamental sit-ups with a 5 second descend.

If you completed this workout, head to Newb Group Workout 3 for your next session. If not, stick with this one until you complete it.

Glasses of water drank today: 1-2-3-4-5-6-7-8-9-10

Hours of sleep last night: 1-2-3-4-5-6-7-8-9-10

Diet: junk: junk food—————semi-healthy—————healthy

# Newb Group Workout 3

Welcome to the Newb Group Workout 3.

For this workout, you have 6 sets with 90 seconds of rest between each set.

Remember to focus on proper form throughout your sets.

Sets:

1. 17 sit-ups
2. 17 sit-ups
3. 17 sit-ups
4. 17 sit-ups
5. 17 sit-ups
6. Max out: perform as many sit-ups as you can.

Max reps: _____

If you completed this workout, head to Newb Group Workout 4 for your next session. If not, stick with this one until you complete it.

Glasses of water drank today: 1-2-3-4-5-6-7-8-9-10

Hours of sleep last night: 1-2-3-4-5-6-7-8-9-10

Diet: junk: junk food————semi-healthy————healthy

# Newb Group Workout 4

Welcome to the Newb Group Workout 4.

For this workout, you have 6 sets with 60 seconds of rest between each set.

Remember to focus on proper form throughout your sets.

Sets:

1. 19 sit-ups
2. 19 sit-ups
3. 19 sit-ups
4. 19 sit-ups
5. 19 sit-ups
6. 5 fundamental sit-ups with a 5 second descend.

If you completed this workout, head to Newb Group Workout 5 for your next session. If not, stick with this one until you complete it.

Glasses of water drank today: 1-2-3-4-5-6-7-8-9-10

Hours of sleep last night: 1-2-3-4-5-6-7-8-9-10

Diet: junk: junk food—————semi-healthy—————healthy

# Newb Group Workout 5

Welcome to the Newb Group Workout 5.

For this workout, you have 6 sets with 60 seconds of rest between each set.

Remember to focus on proper form throughout your sets.

Sets:

1. 21 sit-ups
2. 21 sit-ups
3. 21 sit-ups
4. 21 sit-ups
5. 21 sit-ups
6. 6 fundamental sit-ups with a 5 second descend.

If you completed this workout, head to Newb Group Workout 6 for your next session. If not, stick with this one until you complete it.

Glasses of water drank today: 1-2-3-4-5-6-7-8-9-10

Hours of sleep last night: 1-2-3-4-5-6-7-8-9-10

Diet: junk: junk food—————semi-healthy—————healthy

# Newb Group Workout 6

Welcome to the Newb Group Workout 6.

For this workout, you have 6 sets with 90 seconds of rest between each set.

Remember to focus on proper form throughout your sets.

Sets:

1. 23 sit-ups
2. 23 sit-ups
3. 23 sit-ups
4. 23 sit-ups
5. 23 sit-ups
6. Max out: perform as many sit-ups as you can.

Max reps: _____

Since this is the end of a two-week period, it is time to redo your sit-up assessment to check your progress if you fully completed this workout.

Rest a day and give the assessment a go to see which Group you will be in next.

Glasses of water drank today: 1-2-3-4-5-6-7-8-9-10

Hours of sleep last night: 1-2-3-4-5-6-7-8-9-10

Diet: junk: junk food—————semi-healthy—————healthy

# Greenhorn Group Workouts

# Greenhorn Group Workout 1

Welcome to the Greenhorn Group Workout 1.

For this workout, you have 6 sets with 60 seconds of rest between each set.

Remember to focus on proper form throughout your sets.

Sets:

1. 19 sit-ups
2. 19 sit-ups
3. 19 sit-ups
4. 19 sit-ups
5. 19 sit-ups
6. 4 fundamental sit-ups with a 5 second descend.

If you completed this workout, head to Greenhorn Group Workout 2 for your next session. If not, stick with this one until you complete it.

Glasses of water drank today: 1-2-3-4-5-6-7-8-9-10

Hours of sleep last night: 1-2-3-4-5-6-7-8-9-10

Diet: junk: junk food—————semi-healthy—————healthy

# Greenhorn Group Workout 2

Welcome to the Greenhorn Group Workout 2.

For this workout, you have 6 sets with 60 seconds of rest between each set.

Remember to focus on proper form throughout your sets.

Sets:

1. 20 sit-ups
2. 20 sit-ups
3. 20 sit-ups
4. 20 sit-ups
5. 20 sit-ups
6. 6 fundamental sit-ups with a 5 second descend.

If you completed this workout, head to Greenhorn Group Workout 3 for your next session. If not, stick with this one until you complete it.

Glasses of water drank today: 1-2-3-4-5-6-7-8-9-10

Hours of sleep last night: 1-2-3-4-5-6-7-8-9-10

Diet: junk: junk food—————semi-healthy—————healthy

# Greenhorn Group Workout 3

Welcome to the Greenhorn Group Workout 3.

For this workout, you have 6 sets with 90 seconds of rest between each set.

Remember to focus on proper form throughout your sets.

Sets:

1. 23 sit-ups
2. 23 sit-ups
3. 23 sit-ups
4. 23 sit-ups
5. 23 sit-ups
6. Max out: perform as many sit-ups as you can.

Max reps: _____

If you completed this workout, head to Greenhorn Group Workout 4 for your next session. If not, stick with this one until you complete it.

Glasses of water drank today: 1-2-3-4-5-6-7-8-9-10

Hours of sleep last night: 1-2-3-4-5-6-7-8-9-10

Diet: junk: junk food—————semi-healthy—————healthy

# Greenhorn Group Workout 4

Welcome to the Greenhorn Group Workout 4.

For this workout, you have 6 sets with 60 seconds of rest between each set.

Remember to focus on proper form throughout your sets.

Sets:

1. 25 sit-ups
2. 25 sit-ups
3. 25 sit-ups
4. 25 sit-ups
5. 25 sit-ups
6. 7 fundamental sit-ups with a 5 second descend.

If you completed this workout, head to Greenhorn Group Workout 5 for your next session. If not, stick with this one until you complete it.

Glasses of water drank today: 1-2-3-4-5-6-7-8-9-10

Hours of sleep last night: 1-2-3-4-5-6-7-8-9-10

Diet: junk: junk food—————semi-healthy—————healthy

# Greenhorn Group Workout 5

Welcome to the Greenhorn Group Workout 5.

For this workout, you have 6 sets with 60 seconds of rest between each set.

Remember to focus on proper form throughout your sets.

Sets:

1. 28 sit-ups
2. 28 sit-ups
3. 28 sit-ups
4. 28 sit-ups
5. 28 sit-ups
6. 8 fundamental sit-ups with a 5 second descend.

If you completed this workout, head to Greenhorn Group Workout 6 for your next session. If not, stick with this one until you complete it.

Glasses of water drank today: 1-2-3-4-5-6-7-8-9-10

Hours of sleep last night: 1-2-3-4-5-6-7-8-9-10

Diet: junk: junk food—————semi-healthy—————healthy

# Greenhorn Group Workout 6

Welcome to the Greenhorn Group Workout 6.

For this workout, you have 6 sets with 90 seconds of rest between each set.

Remember to focus on proper form throughout your sets.

Sets:

1. 31 sit-ups
2. 31 sit-ups
3. 31 sit-ups
4. 31 sit-ups
5. 31 sit-ups
6. Max out: perform as many sit-ups as you can.

Max reps: _____

Since this is the end of a two-week period, it is time to redo your sit-up assessment to check your progress if you fully completed this workout.

Rest a day and give the assessment a go to see which Group you will be in next.

## GREENHORN GROUP WORKOUT 6

Glasses of water drank today: 1-2-3-4-5-6-7-8-9-10

Hours of sleep last night: 1-2-3-4-5-6-7-8-9-10

Diet: junk: junk food—————semi-healthy—————healthy

# Cub Group Workouts

# Cub Group Workout 1

Welcome to the Cub Group Workout 1.

For this workout, you have 6 sets with 60 seconds of rest between each set.

Remember to focus on proper form throughout your sets.

Sets:

1. 23 sit-ups
2. 23 sit-ups
3. 23 sit-ups
4. 23 sit-ups
5. 23 sit-ups
6. 2 fundamental sit-ups with a 10 second descend.

If you completed this workout, head to Cub Group Workout 2 for your next session. If not, stick with this one until you complete it.

Glasses of water drank today: 1-2-3-4-5-6-7-8-9-10

Hours of sleep last night: 1-2-3-4-5-6-7-8-9-10

Diet: junk: junk food—————semi-healthy—————healthy

# Cub Group Workout 2

Welcome to the Cub Group Workout 2.

For this workout, you have 6 sets with 60 seconds of rest between each set.

Remember to focus on proper form throughout your sets.

Sets:

1. 25 sit-ups
2. 25 sit-ups
3. 25 sit-ups
4. 25 sit-ups
5. 25 sit-ups
6. 3 fundamental sit-ups with a 10 second descend.

If you completed this workout, head to Cub Group Workout 3 for your next session. If not, stick with this one until you complete it.

Glasses of water drank today: 1-2-3-4-5-6-7-8-9-10

Hours of sleep last night: 1-2-3-4-5-6-7-8-9-10

Diet: junk: junk food—————semi-healthy—————healthy

## Cub Group Workout 3

Welcome to the Cub Group Workout 3.

For this workout, you have 6 sets with 90 seconds of rest between each set.

Remember to focus on proper form throughout your sets.

Sets:

1. 28 sit-ups
2. 28 sit-ups
3. 28 sit-ups
4. 28 sit-ups
5. 28 sit-ups
6. Max out: perform as many sit-ups as you can.

Max reps: _____

If you completed this workout, head to Cub Group Workout 4 for your next session. If not, stick with this one until you complete it.

Glasses of water drank today: 1-2-3-4-5-6-7-8-9-10

Hours of sleep last night: 1-2-3-4-5-6-7-8-9-10

Diet: junk: junk food—————semi-healthy—————healthy

# Cub Group Workout 4

Welcome to the Cub Group Workout 4.

For this workout, you have 6 sets with 60 seconds of rest between each set.

Remember to focus on proper form throughout your sets.

Sets:

1. 31 sit-ups
2. 31 sit-ups
3. 31 sit-ups
4. 31 sit-ups
5. 31 sit-ups
6. 4 fundamental sit-ups with a 10 second descend.

If you completed this workout, head to Cub Group Workout 5 for your next session. If not, stick with this one until you complete it.

Glasses of water drank today: 1-2-3-4-5-6-7-8-9-10

Hours of sleep last night: 1-2-3-4-5-6-7-8-9-10

Diet: junk: junk food—————semi-healthy—————healthy

# Cub Group Workout 5

Welcome to the Cub Group Workout 5.

For this workout, you have 6 sets with 60 seconds of rest between each set.

Remember to focus on proper form throughout your sets.

Sets:

1. 34 sit-ups
2. 34 sit-ups
3. 34 sit-ups
4. 34 sit-ups
5. 34 sit-ups
6. 4 fundamental sit-ups with a 10 second descend.

If you completed this workout, head to Cub Group Workout 6 for your next session. If not, stick with this one until you complete it.

Glasses of water drank today: 1-2-3-4-5-6-7-8-9-10

Hours of sleep last night: 1-2-3-4-5-6-7-8-9-10

Diet: junk: junk food—————semi-healthy—————healthy

# Cub Group Workout 6

Welcome to the Cub Group Workout 6.

For this workout, you have 6 sets with 90 seconds of rest between each set.

Remember to focus on proper form throughout your sets.

Sets:

1. 37 sit-ups
2. 37 sit-ups
3. 37 sit-ups
4. 37 sit-ups
5. 37 sit-ups
6. Max out: perform as many sit-ups as you can.

Max reps: _____

Since this is the end of a two-week period, it is time to redo your sit-up assessment to check your progress if you fully completed this workout.

Rest a day and give the assessment a go to see which Group you will be in next.

Glasses of water drank today: 1-2-3-4-5-6-7-8-9-10

Hours of sleep last night: 1-2-3-4-5-6-7-8-9-10

Diet: junk: junk food—————semi-healthy—————healthy

# Rookie Group Workouts

# Rookie Group Workout 1

Welcome to the Rookie Group Workout 1.

For this workout, you have 6 sets with 60 seconds of rest between each set.

Remember to focus on proper form throughout your sets.

Sets:

1. 28 sit-ups
2. 28 sit-ups
3. 28 sit-ups
4. 28 sit-ups
5. 28 sit-ups
6. 4 fundamental sit-ups with a 10 second descend.

If you completed this workout, head to Cub Group Workout 2 for your next session. If not, stick with this one until you complete it.

Glasses of water drank today: 1-2-3-4-5-6-7-8-9-10

Hours of sleep last night: 1-2-3-4-5-6-7-8-9-10

Diet: junk: junk food—————semi-healthy—————healthy

# Rookie Group Workout 2

Welcome to the Rookie Group Workout 2.

For this workout, you have 6 sets with 60 seconds of rest between each set.

Remember to focus on proper form throughout your sets.

Sets:

1. 31 sit-ups
2. 31 sit-ups
3. 31 sit-ups
4. 31 sit-ups
5. 31 sit-ups
6. 4 fundamental sit-ups with a 10 second descend.

If you completed this workout, head to Rookie Group Workout 3 for your next session. If not, stick with this one until you complete it.

Glasses of water drank today: 1-2-3-4-5-6-7-8-9-10

Hours of sleep last night: 1-2-3-4-5-6-7-8-9-10

Diet: junk: junk food—————semi-healthy—————healthy

# Rookie Group Workout 3

Welcome to the Rookie Group Workout 3.

For this workout, you have 6 sets with 90 seconds of rest between each set.

Remember to focus on proper form throughout your sets.

Sets:

1. 34 sit-ups
2. 34 sit-ups
3. 34 sit-ups
4. 34 sit-ups
5. 34 sit-ups
6. Max out: perform as many sit-ups as you can.

Max reps: _____

If you completed this workout, head to Rookie Group Workout 4 for your next session. If not, stick with this one until you complete it.

Glasses of water drank today: 1-2-3-4-5-6-7-8-9-10

Hours of sleep last night: 1-2-3-4-5-6-7-8-9-10

Diet: junk: junk food—————semi-healthy—————healthy

# Rookie Group Workout 4

Welcome to the Rookie Group Workout 4.

For this workout, you have 6 sets with 60 seconds of rest between each set.

Remember to focus on proper form throughout your sets.

Sets:

1. 37 sit-ups
2. 37 sit-ups
3. 37 sit-ups
4. 37 sit-ups
5. 37 sit-ups
6. 6 fundamental sit-ups with a 10 second descend.

If you completed this workout, head to Rookie Group Workout 5 for your next session. If not, stick with this one until you complete it.

Glasses of water drank today: 1-2-3-4-5-6-7-8-9-10

Hours of sleep last night: 1-2-3-4-5-6-7-8-9-10

Diet: junk: junk food—————semi-healthy—————healthy

# Rookie Group Workout 5

Welcome to the Rookie Group Workout 5.

For this workout, you have 6 sets with 60 seconds of rest between each set.

Remember to focus on proper form throughout your sets.

Sets:

1. 44 sit-ups
2. 44 sit-ups
3. 44 sit-ups
4. 44 sit-ups
5. 44 sit-ups
6. 7 fundamental sit-ups with a 10 second descend.

If you completed this workout, head to Rookie Group Workout 6 for your next session. If not, stick with this one until you complete it.

Glasses of water drank today: 1-2-3-4-5-6-7-8-9-10

Hours of sleep last night: 1-2-3-4-5-6-7-8-9-10

Diet: junk: junk food—————semi-healthy—————healthy

# Rookie Group Workout 6

Welcome to the Rookie Group Workout 6.

For this workout, you have 6 sets with 90 seconds of rest between each set.

Remember to focus on proper form throughout your sets.

Sets:

1. 49 sit-ups
2. 49 sit-ups
3. 49 sit-ups
4. 49 sit-ups
5. 49 sit-ups
6. Max out: perform as many sit-ups as you can.

Max reps: _____

Since this is the end of a two-week period, it is time to redo your sit-up assessment to check your progress if you fully completed this workout.

Rest a day and give the assessment a go to see which Group you will be in next.

ROOKIE GROUP WORKOUT 6

Glasses of water drank today: 1-2-3-4-5-6-7-8-9-10

Hours of sleep last night: 1-2-3-4-5-6-7-8-9-10

Diet: junk: junk food—————semi-healthy—————healthy

# Pleb Group Workouts

# Pleb Group Workout 1

Welcome to the Pleb Group Workout 1.

For this workout, you have 6 sets with 60 seconds of rest between each set.

Remember to focus on proper form throughout your sets.

Sets:

1. 34 sit-ups
2. 34 sit-ups
3. 34 sit-ups
4. 34 sit-ups
5. 34 sit-ups
6. 5 fundamental sit-ups with a 10 second descend.

If you completed this workout, head to Pleb Group Workout 2 for your next session. If not, stick with this one until you complete it.

Glasses of water drank today: 1-2-3-4-5-6-7-8-9-10

Hours of sleep last night: 1-2-3-4-5-6-7-8-9-10

Diet: junk: junk food—————semi-healthy—————healthy

# Pleb Group Workout 2

Welcome to the Pleb Group Workout 2.

For this workout, you have 6 sets with 60 seconds of rest between each set.

Remember to focus on proper form throughout your sets.

Sets:

1. 38 sit-ups
2. 38 sit-ups
3. 38 sit-ups
4. 38 sit-ups
5. 38 sit-ups
6. 6 fundamental sit-ups with a 10 second descend.

If you completed this workout, head to Pleb Group Workout 3 for your next session. If not, stick with this one until you complete it.

Glasses of water drank today: 1-2-3-4-5-6-7-8-9-10

Hours of sleep last night: 1-2-3-4-5-6-7-8-9-10

Diet: junk: junk food—————semi-healthy—————healthy

# Pleb Group Workout 3

Welcome to the Pleb Group Workout 3.

For this workout, you have 6 sets with 90 seconds of rest between each set.

Remember to focus on proper form throughout your sets.

Sets:

1. 42 sit-ups
2. 42 sit-ups
3. 42 sit-ups
4. 42 sit-ups
5. 42 sit-ups
6. Max out: perform as many sit-ups as you can.

Max reps: _____

If you completed this workout, head to Pleb Group Workout 4 for your next session. If not, stick with this one until you complete it.

Glasses of water drank today: 1-2-3-4-5-6-7-8-9-10

Hours of sleep last night: 1-2-3-4-5-6-7-8-9-10

Diet: junk: junk food—————semi-healthy—————healthy

# Pleb Group Workout 4

Welcome to the Pleb Group Workout 4.

For this workout, you have 6 sets with 60 seconds of rest between each set.

Remember to focus on proper form throughout your sets.

Sets:

1. 45 sit-ups
2. 45 sit-ups
3. 45 sit-ups
4. 45 sit-ups
5. 45 sit-ups
6. 8 fundamental sit-ups with a 10 second descend.

If you completed this workout, head to Pleb Group Workout 5 for your next session. If not, stick with this one until you complete it.

Glasses of water drank today: 1-2-3-4-5-6-7-8-9-10

Hours of sleep last night: 1-2-3-4-5-6-7-8-9-10

Diet: junk: junk food—————semi-healthy—————healthy

# Pleb Group Workout 5

Welcome to the Pleb Group Workout 5.

For this workout, you have 6 sets with 60 seconds of rest between each set.

Remember to focus on proper form throughout your sets.

Sets:

1. 53 sit-ups
2. 53 sit-ups
3. 53 sit-ups
4. 53 sit-ups
5. 53 sit-ups
6. 9 fundamental sit-ups with a 10 second descend.

If you completed this workout, head to Pleb Group Workout 6 for your next session. If not, stick with this one until you complete it.

Glasses of water drank today: 1-2-3-4-5-6-7-8-9-10

Hours of sleep last night: 1-2-3-4-5-6-7-8-9-10

Diet: junk: junk food—————semi-healthy—————healthy

# Pleb Group Workout 6

Welcome to the Pleb Group Workout 6.

For this workout, you have 6 sets with 90 seconds of rest between each set.

Remember to focus on proper form throughout your sets.

Sets:

1. 61 sit-ups
2. 61 sit-ups
3. 61 sit-ups
4. 61 sit-ups
5. 61 sit-ups
6. Max out: perform as many sit-ups as you can.

Max reps: _____

Since this is the end of a two-week period, it is time to redo your sit-up assessment to check your progress if you fully completed this workout.

Rest a day and give the assessment a go to see which Group you will be in next.

Glasses of water drank today: 1-2-3-4-5-6-7-8-9-10

Hours of sleep last night: 1-2-3-4-5-6-7-8-9-10

Diet: junk: junk food—————semi-healthy—————healthy

# Gorilla Group Workouts

# Gorilla Group Workout 1

Welcome to the Gorilla Group Workout 1.

For this workout, you have 6 sets with 120 seconds of rest between each set.

Remember to focus on proper form throughout your sets.

Sets:

1. 42 sit-ups
2. 42 sit-ups
3. 42 sit-ups
4. 42 sit-ups
5. 42 sit-ups
6. 5 fundamental sit-ups with a 10 second descend.

If you completed this workout, head to Gorilla Group Workout 2 for your next session. If not, stick with this one until you complete it.

Glasses of water drank today: 1-2-3-4-5-6-7-8-9-10

Hours of sleep last night: 1-2-3-4-5-6-7-8-9-10

Diet: junk: junk food—————semi-healthy—————healthy

# Gorilla Group Workout 2

Welcome to the Gorilla Group Workout 2.

For this workout, you have 9 sets with 90 seconds of rest between each set.

Remember to focus on proper form throughout your sets.

Sets:

1. 28 sit-ups
2. 28 sit-ups
3. 28 sit-ups
4. 28 sit-ups
5. 28 sit-ups
6. 28 sit-ups
7. 28 sit-ups
8. 28 sit-ups
9. 6 fundamental sit-ups with a 10 second descend.

If you completed this workout, head to Gorilla Group Workout 3 for your next session. If not, stick with this one until you complete it.

Glasses of water drank today: 1-2-3-4-5-6-7-8-9-10

Hours of sleep last night: 1-2-3-4-5-6-7-8-9-10

Diet: junk: junk food—————semi-healthy—————healthy

# Gorilla Group Workout 3

Welcome to the Gorilla Group Workout 3.

For this workout, you have 9 sets with 90 seconds of rest between each set.

Remember to focus on proper form throughout your sets.

Sets:

1. 30 sit-ups
2. 30 sit-ups
3. 30 sit-ups
4. 30 sit-ups
5. 30 sit-ups
6. 30 sit-ups
7. 30 sit-ups
8. 30 sit-ups
9. Max out: perform as many sit-ups as you can.

Max reps: _____

If you completed this workout, head to Gorilla Group Workout 4 for your next session. If not, stick with this one until you complete it.

Glasses of water drank today: 1-2-3-4-5-6-7-8-9-10

Hours of sleep last night: 1-2-3-4-5-6-7-8-9-10

Diet: junk: junk food—————semi-healthy—————healthy

# Gorilla Group Workout 4

Welcome to the Gorilla Group Workout 4.

For this workout, you have 6 sets with 120 seconds of rest between each set.

Remember to focus on proper form throughout your sets.

Sets:

1. 61 sit-ups
2. 61 sit-ups
3. 61 sit-ups
4. 61 sit-ups
5. 61 sit-ups
6. 10 fundamental sit-ups with a 10 second descend.

If you completed this workout, head to Gorilla Group Workout 5 for your next session. If not, stick with this one until you complete it.

Glasses of water drank today: 1-2-3-4-5-6-7-8-9-10

Hours of sleep last night: 1-2-3-4-5-6-7-8-9-10

Diet: junk: junk food—————semi-healthy—————healthy

# Gorilla Group Workout 5

Welcome to the Gorilla Group Workout 5.

For this workout, you have 10 sets with 90 seconds of rest between each set.

Remember to focus on proper form throughout your sets.

Sets:

1. 35 sit-ups
2. 35 sit-ups
3. 35 sit-ups
4. 35 sit-ups
5. 35 sit-ups
6. 35 sit-ups
7. 35 sit-ups
8. 35 sit-ups
9. 35 sit-ups
10. 11 fundamental sit-ups with a 10 second descend.

If you completed this workout, head to Gorilla Group Workout 6 for your next session. If not, stick with this one until you complete it.

Glasses of water drank today: 1-2-3-4-5-6-7-8-9-10

## GORILLA GROUP WORKOUT 5

Hours of sleep last night: 1-2-3-4-5-6-7-8-9-10

Diet: junk: junk food—————semi-healthy—————healthy

# Gorilla Group Workout 6

Welcome to the Gorilla Group Workout 6.

For this workout, you have 10 sets with 90 seconds of rest between each set.

Remember to focus on proper form throughout your sets.

Sets:

1. 37 sit-ups
2. 37 sit-ups
3. 37 sit-ups
4. 37 sit-ups
5. 37 sit-ups
6. 37 sit-ups
7. 37 sit-ups
8. 37 sit-ups
9. 37 sit-ups
10. Max out: perform as many sit-ups as you can.

Max reps: _____

Since this is the end of a two-week period, it is time to redo your sit-up assessment to check your progress if you fully completed this workout.

## GORILLA GROUP WORKOUT 6

Rest a day and give the assessment a go to see which Group you will be in next.

Glasses of water drank today: 1-2-3-4-5-6-7-8-9-10

Hours of sleep last night: 1-2-3-4-5-6-7-8-9-10

Diet: junk: junk food —————semi-healthy—————healthy

# Viking Group Workouts

# Viking Group Workout 1

Welcome to the Viking Group Workout 1.

For this workout, you have 6 sets with 120 seconds of rest between each set.

Remember to focus on proper form throughout your sets.

Sets:

1. 56 sit-ups
2. 56 sit-ups
3. 56 sit-ups
4. 56 sit-ups
5. 56 sit-ups
6. 8 fundamental sit-ups with a 10 second descend.

If you completed this workout, head to Viking Group Workout 2 for your next session. If not, stick with this one until you complete it.

Glasses of water drank today: 1-2-3-4-5-6-7-8-9-10

Hours of sleep last night: 1-2-3-4-5-6-7-8-9-10

Diet: junk: junk food—————semi-healthy—————healthy

# Viking Group Workout 2

Welcome to the Viking Group Workout 2.

For this workout, you have 9 sets with 90 seconds of rest between each set.

Remember to focus on proper form throughout your sets.

Sets:

1. 35 sit-ups
2. 35 sit-ups
3. 35 sit-ups
4. 35 sit-ups
5. 35 sit-ups
6. 35 sit-ups
7. 35 sit-ups
8. 35 sit-ups
9. 10 fundamental sit-ups with a 10 second descend.

If you completed this workout, head to Viking Group Workout 3 for your next session. If not, stick with this one until you complete it.

Glasses of water drank today: 1-2-3-4-5-6-7-8-9-10

## VIKING GROUP WORKOUT 2

Hours of sleep last night: 1-2-3-4-5-6-7-8-9-10

Diet: junk: junk food—————semi-healthy—————healthy

# Viking Group Workout 3

Welcome to the Viking Group Workout 3.

For this workout, you have 9 sets with 90 seconds of rest between each set.

Remember to focus on proper form throughout your sets.

Sets:

1. 37 sit-ups
2. 37 sit-ups
3. 37 sit-ups
4. 37 sit-ups
5. 37 sit-ups
6. 37 sit-ups
7. 37 sit-ups
8. 37 sit-ups
9. Max out: perform as many sit-ups as you can.

Max reps: _____

If you completed this workout, head to Viking Group Workout 4 for your next session. If not, stick with this one until you complete it.

VIKING GROUP WORKOUT 3

Glasses of water drank today: 1-2-3-4-5-6-7-8-9-10

Hours of sleep last night: 1-2-3-4-5-6-7-8-9-10

Diet: junk: junk food—————semi-healthy—————healthy

# Viking Group Workout 4

Welcome to the Viking Group Workout 4.

For this workout, you have 6 sets with 120 seconds of rest between each set.

Remember to focus on proper form throughout your sets.

Sets:

1. 70 sit-ups
2. 70 sit-ups
3. 70 sit-ups
4. 70 sit-ups
5. 70 sit-ups
6. 12 fundamental sit-ups with a 10 second descend.

If you completed this workout, head to Viking Group Workout 5 for your next session. If not, stick with this one until you complete it.

Glasses of water drank today: 1-2-3-4-5-6-7-8-9-10

Hours of sleep last night: 1-2-3-4-5-6-7-8-9-10

Diet: junk: junk food———––semi-healthy—––––healthy

# Viking Group Workout 5

Welcome to the Viking Group Workout 5.

For this workout, you have 10 sets with 90 seconds of rest between each set.

Remember to focus on proper form throughout your sets.

Sets:

1. 41 sit-ups
2. 41 sit-ups
3. 41 sit-ups
4. 41 sit-ups
5. 41 sit-ups
6. 41 sit-ups
7. 41 sit-ups
8. 41 sit-ups
9. 41 sit-ups
10. 13 fundamental sit-ups with a 10 second descend.

If you completed this workout, head to Viking Group Workout 6 for your next session. If not, stick with this one until you complete it.

Glasses of water drank today: 1-2-3-4-5-6-7-8-9-10

Hours of sleep last night: 1-2-3-4-5-6-7-8-9-10

Diet: junk: junk food—————semi-healthy—————healthy

# Viking Group Workout 6

Welcome to the Viking Group Workout 6.

For this workout, you have 10 sets with 90 seconds of rest between each set.

Remember to focus on proper form throughout your sets.

Sets:

1. 48 sit-ups
2. 48 sit-ups
3. 48 sit-ups
4. 48 sit-ups
5. 48 sit-ups
6. 48 sit-ups
7. 48 sit-ups
8. 48 sit-ups
9. 48 sit-ups
10. Max out: perform as many sit-ups as you can.

Max reps: _____

Since this is the end of a two-week period, it is time to redo your sit-ups assessment to check your progress if you fully completed this workout.

Rest a day and give the assessment a go to see which Group you will be in next.

Glasses of water drank today: 1-2-3-4-5-6-7-8-9-10

Hours of sleep last night: 1-2-3-4-5-6-7-8-9-10

Diet: junk: junk food—————semi-healthy—————healthy

# Elite Group Workouts

# Elite Group Workout 1

Welcome to the Elite Group Workout 1.

For this workout, you have 6 sets with 120 seconds of rest between each set.

Remember to focus on proper form throughout your sets.

Sets:

1. 66 sit-ups
2. 66 sit-ups
3. 66 sit-ups
4. 66 sit-ups
5. 66 sit-ups
6. 10 fundamental sit-ups with a 10 second descend.

If you completed this workout, head to Elite Group Workout 3 for your next session. If not, stick with this one until you complete it.

Glasses of water drank today: 1-2-3-4-5-6-7-8-9-10

Hours of sleep last night: 1-2-3-4-5-6-7-8-9-10

Diet: junk: junk food—————semi-healthy—————healthy

# Elite Group Workout 2

Welcome to the Elite Group Workout 2.

For this workout, you have 9 sets with 90 seconds of rest between each set.

Remember to focus on proper form throughout your sets.

Sets:

1. 30 sit-ups
2. 30 sit-ups
3. 30 sit-ups
4. 30 sit-ups
5. 30 sit-ups
6. 30 sit-ups
7. 30 sit-ups
8. 30 sit-ups
9. 11 fundamental sit-ups with a 10 second descend.

If you completed this workout, head to Elite Group Workout 3 for your next session. If not, stick with this one until you complete it.

Glasses of water drank today: 1-2-3-4-5-6-7-8-9-10

Hours of sleep last night: 1-2-3-4-5-6-7-8-9-10

Diet: junk: junk food— — — — —semi-healthy— — — — —healthy

# Elite Group Workout 3

Welcome to the Elite Group Workout 3.

For this workout, you have 9 sets with 90 seconds of rest between each set.

Remember to focus on proper form throughout your sets.

Sets:

1. 43 sit-ups
2. 43 sit-ups
3. 43 sit-ups
4. 43 sit-ups
5. 43 sit-ups
6. 43 sit-ups
7. 43 sit-ups
8. 43 sit-ups
9. Max out: perform as many sit-ups as you can.

Max reps: _____

If you completed this workout, head to Elite Group Workout 4 for your next session. If not, stick with this one until you complete it.

Glasses of water drank today: 1-2-3-4-5-6-7-8-9-10

Hours of sleep last night: 1-2-3-4-5-6-7-8-9-10

Diet: junk: junk food————semi-healthy————healthy

# Elite Group Workout 4

Welcome to the Elite Group Workout 4.

For this workout, you have 6 sets with 120 seconds of rest between each set.

Remember to focus on proper form throughout your sets.

Sets:

1. 83 sit-ups
2. 83 sit-ups
3. 83 sit-ups
4. 83 sit-ups
5. 83 sit-ups
6. 14 fundamental sit-ups with a 10 second descend.

If you completed this workout, head to Elite Group Workout 5 for your next session. If not, stick with this one until you complete it.

Glasses of water drank today: 1-2-3-4-5-6-7-8-9-10

Hours of sleep last night: 1-2-3-4-5-6-7-8-9-10

Diet: junk: junk food—————semi-healthy—————healthy

# Elite Group Workout 5

Welcome to the Elite Group Workout 5.

For this workout, you have 10 sets with 90 seconds of rest between each set.

Remember to focus on proper form throughout your sets.

Sets:

1. 48 sit-ups
2. 48 sit-ups
3. 48 sit-ups
4. 48 sit-ups
5. 48 sit-ups
6. 48 sit-ups
7. 48 sit-ups
8. 48 sit-ups
9. 48 sit-ups
10. 15 fundamental sit-ups with a 10 second descend.

If you completed this workout, head to Elite Group Workout 6 for your next session. If not, stick with this one until you complete it.

Glasses of water drank today: 1-2-3-4-5-6-7-8-9-10

## ELITE GROUP WORKOUT 5

Hours of sleep last night: 1-2-3-4-5-6-7-8-9-10

Diet: junk: junk food—————semi-healthy—————healthy

# Elite Group Workout 6

Welcome to the Elite Group Workout 6.

For this workout, you have 10 sets with 90 seconds of rest between each set.

Remember to focus on proper form throughout your sets.

Sets:

1. 54 sit-ups
2. 54 sit-ups
3. 54 sit-ups
4. 54 sit-ups
5. 54 sit-ups
6. 54 sit-ups
7. 54 sit-ups
8. 54 sit-ups
9. 54 sit-ups
10. Max out: perform as many sit-ups as you can.

Max reps: _____

Since this is the end of a two-week period, it is time to redo your sit-up assessment to check your progress if you fully completed this workout.

## ELITE GROUP WORKOUT 6

Rest a day and give the assessment a go to see which Group you will be in next.

Glasses of water drank today: 1-2-3-4-5-6-7-8-9-10

Hours of sleep last night: 1-2-3-4-5-6-7-8-9-10

Diet: junk: junk food——————semi-healthy——————healthy

# Commando Group Workouts

# Commando Group Workout 1

Welcome to the Commando Group Workout 1.

For this workout, you have 6 sets with 120 seconds of rest between each set.

Remember to focus on proper form throughout your sets.

Sets:

1. 70 sit-ups
2. 70 sit-ups
3. 70 sit-ups
4. 70 sit-ups
5. 70 sit-ups
6. 11 fundamental sit-ups with a 10 second descend.

If you completed this workout, head to Commando Group Workout 2 for your next session. If not, stick with this one until you complete it.

Glasses of water drank today: 1-2-3-4-5-6-7-8-9-10

Hours of sleep last night: 1-2-3-4-5-6-7-8-9-10

Diet: junk: junk food—————semi-healthy—————healthy

# Commando Group Workout 2

Welcome to the Commando Group Workout 2.

For this workout, you have 10 sets with 90 seconds of rest between each set.

Remember to focus on proper form throughout your sets.

Sets:

1. 31 sit-ups
2. 31 sit-ups
3. 31 sit-ups
4. 31 sit-ups
5. 31 sit-ups
6. 31 sit-ups
7. 31 sit-ups
8. 31 sit-ups
9. 31 sit-ups
10. 12 fundamental sit-ups with a 10 second descend.

If you completed this workout, head to Commando Group Workout 3 for your next session. If not, stick with this one until you complete it.

Glasses of water drank today: 1-2-3-4-5-6-7-8-9-10

## COMMANDO GROUP WORKOUT 2

Hours of sleep last night: 1-2-3-4-5-6-7-8-9-10

Diet: junk: junk food—————semi-healthy—————healthy

# Commando Group Workout 3

Welcome to the Commando Group Workout 3.

For this workout, you have 10 sets with 90 seconds of rest between each set.

Remember to focus on proper form throughout your sets.

Sets:

1. 46 sit-ups
2. 46 sit-ups
3. 46 sit-ups
4. 46 sit-ups
5. 46 sit-ups
6. 46 sit-ups
7. 46 sit-ups
8. 46 sit-ups
9. 46 sit-ups
10. Max out: perform as many sit-ups as you can.

Max reps: _____

If you completed this workout, head to Commando Group Workout 4 for your next session. If not, stick with this one until you complete it.

## COMMANDO GROUP WORKOUT 3

Glasses of water drank today: 1-2-3-4-5-6-7-8-9-10

Hours of sleep last night: 1-2-3-4-5-6-7-8-9-10

Diet: junk: junk food—————semi-healthy—————healthy

# Commando Group Workout 4

Welcome to the Commando Group Workout 4.

For this workout, you have 6 sets with 120 seconds of rest between each set.

Remember to focus on proper form throughout your sets.

Sets:

1. 86 sit-ups
2. 86 sit-ups
3. 86 sit-ups
4. 86 sit-ups
5. 86 sit-ups
6. 13 fundamental sit-ups with a 10 second descend.

If you completed this workout, head to Commando Group Workout 5 for your next session. If not, stick with this one until you complete it.

Glasses of water drank today: 1-2-3-4-5-6-7-8-9-10

Hours of sleep last night: 1-2-3-4-5-6-7-8-9-10

Diet: junk: junk food—————semi-healthy—————healthy

# Commando Group Workout 5

Welcome to the Commando Group Workout 5.

For this workout, you have 10 sets with 90 seconds of rest between each set.

Remember to focus on proper form throughout your sets.

Sets:

1. 52 sit-ups
2. 52 sit-ups
3. 52 sit-ups
4. 52 sit-ups
5. 52 sit-ups
6. 52 sit-ups
7. 52 sit-ups
8. 52 sit-ups
9. 52 sit-ups
10. 14 fundamental sit-ups with a 10 second descend.

If you completed this workout, head to Commando Group Workout 6 for your next session. If not, stick with this one until you complete it.

Glasses of water drank today: 1-2-3-4-5-6-7-8-9-10

Hours of sleep last night: 1-2-3-4-5-6-7-8-9-10

Diet: junk: junk food—————semi-healthy—————healthy

# Commando Group Workout 6

Welcome to the Commando Group Workout 6.

For this workout, you have 10 sets with 90 seconds of rest between each set.

Remember to focus on proper form throughout your sets.

Sets:

1. 58 sit-ups
2. 58 sit-ups
3. 58 sit-ups
4. 58 sit-ups
5. 58 sit-ups
6. 58 sit-ups
7. 58 sit-ups
8. 58 sit-ups
9. 58 sit-ups
10. Max out: perform as many sit-ups as you can.

Max reps: _____

If you completed this workout, you have earned the right to attempt hitting 200 consecutive sit-ups. Take a few days off to fully recover and take a shot

at hitting your goal.

You got this.

Glasses of water drank today: 1-2-3-4-5-6-7-8-9-10

Hours of sleep last night: 1-2-3-4-5-6-7-8-9-10

Diet: junk: junk food—————semi-healthy—————healthy

# Veteran Group Workouts

# Veteran Group Workout 1

Welcome to the Veteran Group Workout 1.

For this workout, you have 6 sets with 120 seconds of rest between each set.

Remember to focus on proper form throughout your sets.

Sets:

1. 86 sit-ups
2. 86 sit-ups
3. 86 sit-ups
4. 86 sit-ups
5. 86 sit-ups
6. 14 fundamental sit-ups with a 10 second descend.

If you completed this workout, head to Veteran Group Workout 2 for your next session. If not, stick with this one until you complete it.

Glasses of water drank today: 1-2-3-4-5-6-7-8-9-10

Hours of sleep last night: 1-2-3-4-5-6-7-8-9-10

Diet: junk: junk food—————semi-healthy—————healthy

# Veteran Group Workout 2

Welcome to the Veteran Group Workout 2.

For this workout, you have 10 sets with 90 seconds of rest between each set.

Remember to focus on proper form throughout your sets.

Sets:

1. 45 sit-ups
2. 45 sit-ups
3. 45 sit-ups
4. 45 sit-ups
5. 45 sit-ups
6. 45 sit-ups
7. 45 sit-ups
8. 45 sit-ups
9. 45 sit-ups
10. 15 fundamental sit-ups with a 10 second descend.

If you completed this workout, head to Veteran Group Workout 3 for your next session. If not, stick with this one until you complete it.

Glasses of water drank today: 1-2-3-4-5-6-7-8-9-10

Hours of sleep last night: 1-2-3-4-5-6-7-8-9-10

Diet: junk: junk food—————semi-healthy—————healthy

# Veteran Group Workout 3

Welcome to the Veteran Group Workout 3.

For this workout, you have 10 sets with 90 seconds of rest between each set.

Remember to focus on proper form throughout your sets.

Sets:

1. 52 sit-ups
2. 52 sit-ups
3. 52 sit-ups
4. 52 sit-ups
5. 52 sit-ups
6. 52 sit-ups
7. 52 sit-ups
8. 52 sit-ups
9. 52 sit-ups
10. Max out: perform as many sit-ups as you can.

Max reps: _____

If you completed this workout, head to Veteran Group Workout 4 for your next session. If not, stick with this one until you complete it.

Glasses of water drank today: 1-2-3-4-5-6-7-8-9-10

Hours of sleep last night: 1-2-3-4-5-6-7-8-9-10

Diet: junk: junk food—————semi-healthy—————healthy

# Veteran Group Workout 4

Welcome to the Veteran Group Workout 4.

For this workout, you have 6 sets with 120 seconds of rest between each set.

Remember to focus on proper form throughout your sets.

Sets:

1. 106 sit-ups
2. 106 sit-ups
3. 106 sit-ups
4. 106 sit-ups
5. 106 sit-ups
6. 16 fundamental sit-ups with a 10 second descend.

If you completed this workout, head to Veteran Group Workout 5 for your next session. If not, stick with this one until you complete it.

Glasses of water drank today: 1-2-3-4-5-6-7-8-9-10

Hours of sleep last night: 1-2-3-4-5-6-7-8-9-10

Diet: junk: junk food—————semi-healthy—————healthy

# Veteran Group Workout 5

Welcome to the Veteran Group Workout 5.

For this workout, you have 10 sets with 90 seconds of rest between each set.

Remember to focus on proper form throughout your sets.

Sets:

1. 58 sit-ups
2. 58 sit-ups
3. 58 sit-ups
4. 58 sit-ups
5. 58 sit-ups
6. 58 sit-ups
7. 58 sit-ups
8. 58 sit-ups
9. 58 sit-ups
10. 17 fundamental sit-ups with a 10 second descend.

If you completed this workout, head to Veteran Group Workout 6 for your next session. If not, stick with this one until you complete it.

Glasses of water drank today: 1-2-3-4-5-6-7-8-9-10

## VETERAN GROUP WORKOUT 5

Hours of sleep last night: 1-2-3-4-5-6-7-8-9-10

Diet: junk: junk food—————semi-healthy—————healthy

# Veteran Group Workout 6

Welcome to the Veteran Group Workout 6.

For this workout, you have 10 sets with 90 seconds of rest between each set.

Remember to focus on proper form throughout your sets.

Sets:

1. 66 sit-ups
2. 66 sit-ups
3. 66 sit-ups
4. 66 sit-ups
5. 66 sit-ups
6. 66 sit-ups
7. 66 sit-ups
8. 66 sit-ups
9. 66 sit-ups
10. Max out: perform as many sit-ups as you can.

Max reps: _____

If you completed this workout, you have earned the right to attempt hitting 200 consecutive sit-ups. Take a few days off to fully recover and take a shot

## VETERAN GROUP WORKOUT 6

at hitting your goal.

You got this.

Glasses of water drank today: 1-2-3-4-5-6-7-8-9-10

Hours of sleep last night: 1-2-3-4-5-6-7-8-9-10

Diet: junk: junk food—————semi-healthy—————healthy

# Nuclear Group Workouts

# Nuclear Group Workout 1

Welcome to the Nuclear Group Workout 1.

For this workout, you have 6 sets with 120 seconds of rest between each set.

Remember to focus on proper form throughout your sets.

Sets:

1. 99 sit-ups
2. 99 sit-ups
3. 99 sit-ups
4. 99 sit-ups
5. 99 sit-ups
6. 15 fundamental sit-ups with a 10 second descend.

If you completed this workout, head to Nuclear Group Workout 2 for your next session. If not, stick with this one until you complete it.

Glasses of water drank today: 1-2-3-4-5-6-7-8-9-10

Hours of sleep last night: 1-2-3-4-5-6-7-8-9-10

Diet: junk: junk food—————semi-healthy—————healthy

# Nuclear Group Workout 2

Welcome to the Nuclear Group Workout 2.

For this workout, you have 10 sets with 90 seconds of rest between each set.

Remember to focus on proper form throughout your sets.

Sets:

1. 52 sit-ups
2. 52 sit-ups
3. 52 sit-ups
4. 52 sit-ups
5. 52 sit-ups
6. 52 sit-ups
7. 52 sit-ups
8. 52 sit-ups
9. 52 sit-ups
10. 16 fundamental sit-ups with a 10 second descend.

If you completed this workout, head to Nuclear Group Workout 3 for your next session. If not, stick with this one until you complete it.

Glasses of water drank today: 1-2-3-4-5-6-7-8-9-10

## NUCLEAR GROUP WORKOUT 2

Hours of sleep last night: 1-2-3-4-5-6-7-8-9-10

Diet: junk: junk food———––semi-healthy———––healthy

# Nuclear Group Workout 3

Welcome to the Nuclear Group Workout 3.

For this workout, you have 10 sets with 90 seconds of rest between each set.

Remember to focus on proper form throughout your sets.

Sets:

1. 58 sit-ups
2. 58 sit-ups
3. 58 sit-ups
4. 58 sit-ups
5. 58 sit-ups
6. 58 sit-ups
7. 58 sit-ups
8. 58 sit-ups
9. 58 sit-ups
10. Max out: perform as many sit-ups as you can.

Max reps: _____

If you completed this workout, head to Nuclear Group Workout 4 for your next session. If not, stick with this one until you complete it.

## NUCLEAR GROUP WORKOUT 3

Glasses of water drank today: 1-2-3-4-5-6-7-8-9-10

Hours of sleep last night: 1-2-3-4-5-6-7-8-9-10

Diet: junk: junk food—————semi-healthy—————healthy

# Nuclear Group Workout 4

Welcome to the Nuclear Group Workout 4.

For this workout, you have 6 sets with 120 seconds of rest between each set.

Remember to focus on proper form throughout your sets.

Sets:

1. 109 sit-ups
2. 109 sit-ups
3. 109 sit-ups
4. 109 sit-ups
5. 109 sit-ups
6. 17 fundamental sit-ups with a 10 second descend.

If you completed this workout, head to Nuclear Group Workout 5 for your next session. If not, stick with this one until you complete it.

Glasses of water drank today: 1-2-3-4-5-6-7-8-9-10

Hours of sleep last night: 1-2-3-4-5-6-7-8-9-10

Diet: junk: junk food—————semi-healthy—————healthy

# Nuclear Group Workout 5

Welcome to the Nuclear Group Workout 5.

For this workout, you have 10 sets with 90 seconds of rest between each set.

Remember to focus on proper form throughout your sets.

Sets:

1. 66 sit-ups
2. 66 sit-ups
3. 66 sit-ups
4. 66 sit-ups
5. 66 sit-ups
6. 66 sit-ups
7. 66 sit-ups
8. 66 sit-ups
9. 66 sit-ups
10. 18 fundamental sit-ups with a 10 second descend.

If you completed this workout, head to Nuclear Group Workout 6 for your next session. If not, stick with this one until you complete it.

Glasses of water drank today: 1-2-3-4-5-6-7-8-9-10

Hours of sleep last night: 1-2-3-4-5-6-7-8-9-10

Diet: junk: junk food————semi-healthy————healthy

# Nuclear Group Workout 6

Welcome to the Nuclear Group Workout 6.

For this workout, you have 10 sets with 90 seconds of rest between each set.

Remember to focus on proper form throughout your sets.

Sets:

1. 70 sit-ups
2. 70 sit-ups
3. 70 sit-ups
4. 70 sit-ups
5. 70 sit-ups
6. 70 sit-ups
7. 70 sit-ups
8. 70 sit-ups
9. 70 sit-ups
10. Max out: perform as many sit-ups as you can.

Max reps: _____

If you completed this workout, you have earned the right to attempt hitting 200 consecutive sit-ups. Take a few days off to fully recover and take a shot

at hitting your goal.

You got this.

Glasses of water drank today: 1-2-3-4-5-6-7-8-9-10

Hours of sleep last night: 1-2-3-4-5-6-7-8-9-10

Diet: junk: junk food—————semi-healthy—————healthy

# Attempting 200 Consecutive Sit-ups

If you are here, that means you have completed either the Commando, Veteran, or Nuclear Group Workouts and have earned the right to attempt nailing down 200 consecutive sit-ups.

This goal is well within your grasp and all you have to do is take it.

As you begin to warm up to crush this, I would like to ask a favor.

I am going to be greedy for a minute here and ask you to leave a review for the book.

Reviews are a pain to get but it will only take a minute or two to leave one.

Scan this QR which will take you straight to the book's page on Amazon.

Scroll down and click the 'leave a customer review' button, select your star rating, leave a few words, and that is it!

It is that simple!

Once that is done, get ready to crush this.

Get psyched for what is about to happen.

Give it everything you have got to knock out as many correct sit-ups without stopping.

Once you are done, come back.

* * *

If you nailed 200 or more, awesome.

That is incredible. Time to knock that off your bucket list.

If you did not quite get it, no worries. Not everyone gets it on the first try.

Use this number as your new assessment number and get back at it!

Cheers.

## Conclusion:

I just want to thank you for making your way through this program and the book. You have bettered yourself for it.

I hope you have challenged yourself and I hope you tasted victory by reaching 200 consecutive sit-ups.

If you are hungry for more challenges, we have got plenty more where this came from.

And if you have enjoyed this book, take a second to leave a review.

Until next time.

Cheers.

Printed in Great Britain
by Amazon